Bull

Quick And Simple Bulletproof Diet Recipes For Weight
Loss, Enhanced Energy, And Radiant Health

*(A Comprehensive Collection Of Numerous Recipes That
Can Be Used While On The Bulletproof Diet)*

Andrzej MacKenzie

TABLE OF CONTENT

Introduction

Will you have oil-infused espresso or tea?

I've heard numerous pessimistic responses to this question, and it's disheartening how much some individuals miss out on the fantastic options and medical benefits available.

I concur that combining oils with coffee and tea appears to be a no-no, but the experience is what is required here. My initial encounter with unrivalled coffee was disastrous. How would you mix margarine with espresso and consume the mixture? I pondered. However, after trying my first cup, I can attest that I have never had espresso without a superior method.

It is stimulating, satiating, and nutrient-dense to help low-carb dieters eat less. Especially when practising intermittent fasting, unbeatable plans are fantastic for keeping you satisfied for a long time. I strongly recommend it.

Therefore, I will discuss thirty intriguing ways to incorporate indestructible into your diet. Whether for breakfast, as an accompaniment to a beverage, or while serving beverages to companions. There is something for every event.

Chapter 1: Should You Adhere To The Bulletproof Diet?

The sense does not affect the weight-lo slam of the bulletrroof rlan, even for long-term weight-lo.

Hghlu retrstve diets, such as the bulletrroof det, mau jumr-tart your weght loss, but they do not uuallu work to keer the weght off because t' shallengng to tau on a diet lke th for an extended period of tme. The key to effective weight loss is finding something you can commit to long-term.

Most nutritionists and dietitians recommend a slow and steady weight loss of one to two pounds per week, which is significantly slower than the one pound per week recommended by the Bulletproof Diet. A usseful det encourages healthy lifestyle changes, such as whole foods, more fruits and vegetables, and increased physical activity; you want to be healthy and maintain your weight loss. Dietary schemes that emphasise rrorretaru rrodust and urrlement should be avoided.

It is strongly discouraged to follow Bulletroof's exercise recommendations. Increasing your daily physical activity is essential, not only for weight loss but also for your health as a whole. In addition to helping you lose weight, exercise can also assist you in maintaining your weight loss, which is your ultimate goal.

Remember that no diet plan is effective for everyone, and no foods or oils will cause you to lose weight. Several factors, including age, gender, activity level, overall health, medications, etc., affect how much weight you gain. If you are unsure of what to do, seek medical advice from your health care provider to develop realistic and healthy weight loss goals.

Anu det rlan that you select should emphasise a lifestyle that you can maintain. This will enable you to simply make permanent changes to your daily eating and exercise habits, resulting in improvements to your health.

Chapter 2: Can It Help You Shed Pounds?

There are no weight loss studies examining the effectiveness of the Bulletproof Diet. According to research, there is no single optimal diet for weight loss. Low-carb, high-fat diets such as the ketogenic diet have been shown to result in more difficult weight loss than other diets, but this difference appears to diminish over time. The best predictor of weight loss is your ability to adhere to a low-calorie diet for an extended period of time. Therefore, the Bulletproof Diet's effect on your weight depends on the number of calories you consume and the length of time you adhere to it. Due to their high fat content, ketogenic diets are satiating and may enable you to eat less and lose weight rapidly. That being said, the Bulletproof Diet does not restrict calories, suggesting that you can achieve a healthy weight by consuming only Bulletproof foods. Yet weight loss is not that difficult. Your weight is influenced by multiple factors, including genetics, physiology, and behaviour. Consequently, regardless of how "Bulletproof" your diet is, you may need to simply make an effort to reduce calorie absorption. You must also adhere to the diet long-term for it to be effective.

Work that could be taxing for some individuals.

The Components of Bulletproofing Your Diet for Rapid Weight Loss

To effectively adhere to a diet plan, you must do your homework and understand it. Knowing why you're doing something not only helps you stick to the plan, but also allows you to customise it so that it works even better with your biochemistry. So, let's take a closer look at the various components that simply make up your diet for shedding fat and regaining health.

Ketogenic

Your bulletproof diet is both low-carb and high-fat, so it is a ketogenic diet. This means that you are reducing your body mass in favour of fuel. Our bodies obtain energy by converting carbohydrates into glucose, which is then metabolised for energy. Whatever isn't used is stored in fat deposits for use when necessary. These are our affection handles. However, your product is fully capable of operating on a higher-octane fuel, ketones. In actuality, newborns are ketogens, and they remain so until they begin receiving carbohydrates. Ketones are produced from dietary fat and provide a great deal of energy without the hormonal fluctuations and cravings that sugar can cause. Just like high-octane gasoline, they burn cleaner and provide greater gas mileage. Why don't we administer ketones to a newborn? Besaue carb conversion lework for your utem, and I'm sorry to say that it can be as difficult as any of u. As long as it contains sufficient carbohydrates, your body will utilise the "carb-to-glucose-to-energy/fat" pathway. Controlling, in fact drastically reducing, the amount of available carbohydrates will allow you to get off the couch and start working. So, a low-carb diet pushes you toward ketosis, a metabolic state in which your body uses ketones as its primary fuel source. However, making ketones requires more fat than we're accustomed to consuming. modern, low-fat society Our dietary fat intake is supplemented by stored body fat in order to provide enough raw material for the production of all ketones. Fat loss, yay! But if you don't consume enough fat and restrict your carbohydrate intake, you have a recipe for disaster. A low-carb diet requires a high-fat diet. Otherwise, our bread is extremely low in sugar and fat and contains FAMINE... It must store as much fat as possible in order to survive the coming hard times. This is the plan of deral manu det. We'd all love to eat sardines and live on rare tyres, but it's impossible unless you're truly starving. Then a multitude of other physical issues, including heart muscle degeneration, join the party. This is the danger associated with anorexia, and you do not wish to go there. To prevent this, you must provide your body with usable fuel in the form of fat. A high fat intake is quite disturbing... And our system does not worry about fuel storage in preparation for a famine. When t needs a little more, it goes to the fat that's stored around your middle and causes you to gain weight. You must eat fat in order to lose fat, as counterintuitive as that may sound. For many roles, eating enough fat to maintain ketosis is a significant barrier to successfully following a low-carb diet. Many people have never consumed full-fat milk, and it may be difficult to break the habit of reaching for low-calorie non-fat yoghurt! The famine/abundance senaro is what causes the phenomenon known as "uo-uo dieting." Your ship had plenty of reclaimed fuel and a substantial amount of weight. When fuel becomes plentiful again, the ship will store as much as possible to prepare for the next attack. The weight is derived from bask (plus some), and o it goes. Your metabolism is constantly on the defensive, torn between family and work, and it can become slowed down by this. A sufficient amount of fat in your diet prevents yo-yo dieting because your brain cannot detect impending famine and your metabolism can function normally. On a long-term ketogenic diet, you can anticipate an average of one round of fat loss per day. That is a great deal of body fat, not actual weight. There are times when your overall weight does not change but your body shape does. As you lose fat and build muscle, you will notice a difference in how your clothes fit, but the bathroom scale may not reflect this.

Intermittent Fasting

Intermittent fasting is simply going without food for a specified period of time. Unless you're reading the newspaper every two hours all night, you're already intermittently fasting... but we are typically not 'sleeping' If you skip breakfast, you are actually eating between 2 0 and 2 6 hours per day. We simply do not typically consider it in this way. Although some diets recommend an alternate-day schedule, the majority of people find that restricting their food intake to a specific period of 6 to 8 hours per day works extremely well for them. Continuous eating by oneself can cause obesity in a number of people. Current research focuses extensively on the health benefits of intermittent fasting. In as little as three weeks, it can help regulate blood sugar, insulin levels, and cholesterol. The risk of sanser eem to be reduced by intermittent fatng and our normal rate of sell deteroration, resulting in an anti-aging effect. One study demonstrated a reduction of up to 8 10 percent in the risk of coronary heart disease, and another demonstrated that regular eating could reduce the risk of developing diabetes and Alzheimer's. These research studies are ongoing, with additional positive findings being released daily. This health benefit is one of the ways you can improve your health with a bulletproof diet, and intermittent fasting is an integral part of the plan. Breakfat is served with high-ostane coffee, which keeps you feeling full until lunch and provides a great deal of energy, but does not metabolise to kick you out of the fed state. You will consume lunch and dinner within a 6- to 8-hour window in the afternoon and evening, and then revert to a fasting state while you sleep.

Anti-Inflammatory:

As a matter of fact, the bulletproof vest originated from fighting fire. Arreu discovered that many of his soreness, swelling, and general malady stemmed from various types of inflammation in his body. He discovered that various natural and synthetic toxins found in food and drink were largely responsible for this inflammation. Through medsal testing, shemsal analysis, and self-experimentation, Arreu bio-hacked the elimination of toxins from his food supply, thereby restoring his sense of health and well-being. Coffee is a good illustration of how the system worked. On some days, coffee energised Asprey and made him feel good; on other days, the same amount of coffee had no positive effect. Could it not be the coffee itself? Uron discovered that some varieties of coffee contained more mould toxins than others. Through self-experimentation, he discovered that the higher the toxin level, the worse it made him feel, so he searched for virtually mold-free coffee. Bingo! He received all of the energising and anti-oxidant benefits of coffee without any negative side effects. Thus, Urgraded Coffee was created. Extensive research revealed additional factors that negatively impact our health in the same manner. Just like the 'beneath' mould toxins found in many foods, not just coffee, there are many natural substances that can have the same effect, causing irritation and inflammation that makes us feel awful. Manu shemsal and artificial additives in processed food appear to produce the same result, as do certain cooking techniques. This is achieved by removing a substantial amount of toxins from the bulletproof diet. The bulletproof diet consists of more than just eating organs, setting it apart from most other eating plans. Certain foods contain substances that, regardless of how they are grown or processed, appear to be persistent irritants and cause chronic inflammation. In general, eliminating them from your diet will improve your health. In addition, our bo-ndvdtu means that each individual's reronal toxins must be identified and eliminated for that individual to enjoy optimal health and well-being. This is the tweaking and customization aspect of becoming bulletproof, where you do your own bulletproofing and experiment with the "freshest" foods.

Timed Eating:

The third component of the bulletproof diet is referred to as timed eating. When consumed too late in the day, coffee can cause a great deal of problems for most roles. Utilizing a food's effect on your body to your advantage is the essence of controlled eating. Carbohydrates are notorious for causing an energy surge followed by a crash. Theu frequently leave you more exhausted than you were before, before they burn off. This is the main issue with a breakfast high in turkey sausage: the mid-morning slump. Being bulletproof involves reserving the majority of your sardines for dinner. You can use your diminishing energy to fall asleep more quickly at night. The downside of sarb immediately became an advantage! High-octane coffee is the opposite of low-octane coffee. You're

19

using the caffeine in that coffee to do what it does best, which is to wake you up and stimulate your mind. Its effects are positive when administered in the morning, and they will be gone by evening, so it will not interfere with your sleep. Timing is of the utmost importance!

Chapter 3: Bulletproof Intermittent Fasting For Weight Loss And Muscle Gain

A biohack that enables fat loss while increasing mental and physical energy without starvation.

You begin the day by consuming a cup of Bulletproof Coffee. The healthy fats provide a steady supply of energy, while the ultra-low-toxin Bulletproof Coffee beans promote lean muscle growth and fat loss. Follow the tor portion of the diet in conjunction with this rrotosol for optimal results.

Bulletproof Proton Fetching

A bohask used ossaonallu to reduce inflammation more effectively.

Approximately once or twice per week, limit your protein intake to 2 10 –210 grammes to help you lose weight without losing muscle. To keep you full and energised throughout the day, consume a cup of Bulletproof Coffee in the morning and a diet high in fats and moderate in carbohydrates. Follow the tor portion of the diet and limit sarbohudrates to the afternoon and evening for optimal results.

Chapter 4: Is Fasting Recommended On The Bulletproof Diet?

True and no. If fasting entails starvation and abstinence from food for days, this is not the case. Instead, the Bulletproof Diet helps you avoid certain foods at specific times so that you can reap the benefits of eating without experiencing an energy crash. Adopt the recommended Bulletproof Roadmap of food (visit www.bulletproof.som/det-roadmap-roter to obtain the Bulletproof Diet Roadmap downloadable roter), use the recipes in this book, and then rrastse two ossaonal ture of fasting to kick-start weight loss, reduce inflammation, detox your body, and accelerate your results.

BULLETPROOF SPORADIC FASTING

Bulletproof Intermittent Fasting requires significantly less willpower than other forms of intermittent fasting. In fact, there is no requirement. This technique is common in biohacking circles because it not only promotes fat loss, but it also builds muscle, combats disease-causing inflammation, and increases your body's resiliency by burning more fat, thereby allowing it to consume less insulin. The main concept behind traditional intermittent fasting is that you consume all of your daily calories within an eight-hour window and then fast for the remainder of the day. Bulletproof Intermittent Fasting, on the other hand, is a fundamentally new and distinct concept that solves the problem of conventional fasting. With conventional eating, you might consume breakfast, lunch at 2 p.m., and dinner before 8 p.m. You wouldn't eat the rest of the day, and you would likely become hungry and weak around 2 2 a.m. if you had a typical job. For people with a significant amount of weight to lose, such as more than 6 0 pounds, fasting can be distracting and hinder mental and physical reconditioning, which is why Bulletproof Intermittent Fasting (see sample day) is a great way to reap the benefits of fasting without the negative side effects.

If you're a busy entrepreneur or a student who relies on mental acuity 28 hours a day, you may find that traditional intermittent fasting leaves you hungry and exhausted at 2 2 a.m., causing your adrenals to work harder to keep your blood sugar stable. By consuming Bulletproof Coffee (with no protein or carbohydrates of any kind) during your "fasting" time, you can experience extreme hunger and full-rower energy while reaping the benefits of an extended fast. The clever thing is that an all-fat breakfast (such as Bulletproof Coffee) won't trick your body into thinking you've broken your fast, so you can reap the benefits of eating without feeling deprived. It's amazing!

Now let's discuss why Bulletproof Intermittent Fasting is superior to conventional intermittent fasting. It's as a result of mTor, a major meshanm that has written itself into our DNA. Both exercise and coffee raise your energy levels while temporarily inhibiting your muscle-building mechanism (the mTor), allowing it to "spring back" and build even more muscle as soon as you eat.

Therefore, in order to build muscle, you must suppress mTor; muscle building occurs when mTor rebounds after being repressed. Therefore, anything that helps you push it down harder will cause it to contract even more forcefully, allowing you to gain muscle. Ways to reduce mTor include intermittent fasting, exercise, and coffee; on sale, chocolate, green tea, turmeric, and resveratrol are also effective. So what then? Bulletproof Intermittent Fasting san simply make your mTor bounse bask. In 2 8 months, despite consuming 8 ,000 calories per day with no exercise, I went from 6 00 pounds to a lean mash-up with a six-pack after experimenting with this concept and figuring out how to maximise my mTor function. Plan intermittent fasting does not use coffee, so it only inhibits one or two of the three problematic mTOR enzymes. Bulletproof Internet Protocol Fasting is more effective because it utilises all three mechanisms: intermittent fasting, exercise, and caffeine.

The following reason for Bulletrroof Intermttent Bulletproof Coffee is superior to traditional intermittent fasting because one of its ingredients increases the point at which you enter ketosis, thereby fueling your brain and enabling you to maintain a ketogenic state despite the presence of carbohydrates in your diet. We use XCT oil, which is effective because it generates molecules known as ketones in the bloodstream. The liver produces ketones from fatty acids during calorie-restricted periods. A momentary spike in these ketone induces hunger, so while fats such as coconut oil and regular MCT oil do not spike it enough to feel the full effect, XCT oil takes on the challenge because it contains C8 and C2 0, the ideal combination of fatty acids. It produces ketones because fat is metabolised differently than carbohydrates, and certain parts of the brain prefer fuel derived from fat over glucose.

For these reasons, it only makes sense to add Bulletproof to the list. Caffeine for the situation. A Bulletproof Intermttent is much simpler and more rleaant to execute. A faster fast than a rlan.

Chapter 5: The Reality Behind Frequent Dietary Myths

Your body requires five things in order for you to lose weight on any diet: energy for your brain, fuel to help drive your body, nutrients for your body cells, the absence of toxins that are unnecessarily harming your body, and a feeling of satiety throughout the day. In actuality, many of these popular "diets" contribute to the obesity epidemic rather than assisting individuals in losing weight.

These diets also contribute to the propagation of numerous popular diet myths. In this chapter, we will examine five of the most pervasive industry myths and then examine the Bulletproof perspective on each.

Myth 2 : If you are not losing weight, you are not trying hard enough.

This is one of the myths that tends to cause the most harm, as it affects a large number of people who are currently struggling with their weight. It is not as if these people are unaware of their states, given that the information is shoved down their throats daily.

The issue is not that these individuals are unaware of the health of their bodies; rather, they are losing a daily battle of will against their bodies' biological need for food. It also does not help that neither society nor medical professionals recognise this. Most physicians and members of modern society misunderstand the power of will and believe that the only way to lose weight is to refuse to eat.

What these doctors and others do not comprehend is that we do not possess an infinite supply of willpower. It is entirely possible to lose one's willpower, and the vast majority of obese individuals have done so long before deciding to seek help.

This phenomenon is known as decision fatigue, and it is the primary reason you simply make poor diet decisions and lose the willpower to select a food that is ultimately more satisfying and healthier for you.

Second Fallacy: You are not as hungry as you believe you are.

It is true that hunger not only improves performance, but also saps energy and makes people irritable and unproductive. Additionally, it is responsible for diminishing your willpower.

In all honesty, hunger is an enormous waste of time. It diverts your attention away from important matters and increases the likelihood that you will simply make more errors than usual.

The Bulletproof diet essentially hacks your appetite by balancing the hormones that control this fundamental function, such as Leptin and Ghrelin.

Everyone acknowledges that hunger is difficult to ignore. Nonetheless, it is entirely manageable so long as you resist your food cravings. By adhering to this diet, you will be able to exert control over your natural biology and no longer be distracted by hunger.

Myth 6 : The only healthy type of diet is a low-fat diet.

Since the 2 910 0s, food chemists have been developing a variety of low-fat foods to combat heart disease.

Nevertheless, when fat is removed from food, only protein and sugar remain. To maintain the integrity of this food, you must replace the fat with something else. Unfortunately, the majority of food chemists insisted on substituting sugar for a healthier alternative.

One of the primary reasons why dieters fail is that they feel tortured by the inability to consume filling and satisfying foods. You do not have to endure such hardships on the Bulletproof diet, as you will have the opportunity to consume extremely scrumptious and satiating foods.

Fat is one of the primary building blocks of the Bulletproof diet, which can be incredibly nourishing if you use the correct fat sources. These fat sources will leave you feeling extremely satisfied, which will aid your diet adherence over the long term.

Myth No. 10 : The only way to lose weight is by cutting calories as much as possible.

If you are the type of person who believes that calories rather than fat consumption are the reason why people gain weight today, you will be surprised. The reality is that it makes no difference how many calories you consume. In fact, your brain uses up to 210 percent of the total calories you consume daily. In light of this, you can consume as many calories as you like without worrying about gaining weight.

While reducing calories may help you lose a little bit of weight, there are many other factors that contribute to weight loss, such as the room temperature, the amount of sleep you get, and even how hard you breathe.

As soon as you stop focusing on how many calories you consume daily, you will be able to pay more attention to the quality of the food you eat in order to provide your body with the proper nutrition it requires.

Chapter 6 : The Deadliest Error In Muscle Building Exposed

What is the most fatal error that will negatively impact the results of fast muscle gain workout techniques? Overtraining is one of the most dangerous yet frequently overlooked muscle-building mistakes, and every workout participant will experience it at least once.

Overtraining is a greater issue than it initially appears because it can severely harm your health. Your muscles can become severely injured, and you can also experience chronic fatigue or muscle loss. Even seasoned bodybuilders are sometimes victims of overtraining because many bodybuilders believe that excessive training can result in rapid muscle growth.

It doesn't matter what kind of fitness goal you have; in order to gain muscle, you must work extremely hard. This is because you're aiming to add mass to your body, which is only possible through intense exercise.

However, due to genetic differences, what may work for a professional bodybuilder may not work for us. Progressive training is essential for rapid muscle gain; you must gradually overload your muscles by increasing the intensity of weight-based exercise programmes.

There are two important factors to consider: ensuring adequate rest between workouts and a gradual increase in intensity. We are typically impatient, and as soon as they determine that we can lift a particular dumbbell, they move on to a heavier one without realising that they are straining our muscles.

Analyzing your improvements is the only way to ensure that you are gaining muscle quickly through progressive training. For example, if you can perform 8 0 push-ups this week and 10 0 the following week, you are following progressive training, whereas if you can perform 10 0 this week and 8 0 next week, you probably need to rest.

Before resuming your workouts, you must ensure that you have fully recovered from your dizziness, regardless of how long it takes you to feel normal again.

Chapter 7: How Can Overtraining Be Avoided?

By determining the optimal workout volume, one can prevent overtraining. You must determine the appropriate amount of weight to lift and the number of repetitions required. The greatest obstacle is that you are the only person who can determine your potential, and judging it on your own at first can be quite difficult.

One of the most common errors individuals simply make is continuing to exercise with injured muscles. You are likely continuing your workout with a lower intensity, but the best way to recover from an injury and gain muscle quickly is to wait until you are completely healed. This may sound challenging, but it is the only viable option!

40

Nutrition is another important aspect of gaining muscle quickly; in fact, it is the most important factor in gaining muscle quickly. You must adhere to a nutrient-dense, yet simple, diet plan every day and avoid skipping meals, especially breakfast.

Ensure you eat whenever you feel hungry, or your muscle tissue will be broken down. If you are not trying to lose weight, you should eat before your workouts. If you can adhere to these rules, gaining muscle quickly is not an impossible task, and you can build muscle relatively quickly.

Chapter 8: Permanently Bulletproof

In maintenance mode, you will achieve the best results if you adhere as closely as possible to the diet's fundamental principles. Bulletproof Coffee and Intermittent Fasting should be consumed daily. Perform the fast once a week and avoid unhealthy foods as much as possible. The primary difference during maintenance mode is whether test foods are consumed or not. This is entirely dependent on how you respond to these foods. During the two-week protocol, the following foods were evaluated. When you are aware of the foods to which you are sensitive, you can simply make the best choices for yourself, your body, and the performance of your body.

Evening carbohydrate intake can be increased if desired. Simply shorten your pants if they have become too snug. Even if you wanted to, you could consume carbohydrates in the morning. You are aware that your body is resilient and able to manage the situation.

During maintenance mode, if it makes you feel better, you may consume something other than coffee for breakfast. Don't forget to practise intermittent fasting occasionally.

You may occasionally consume unhealthy foods, but keep in mind that you may feel ill for one or two days afterwards. Minor modifications are permissible and do not indicate failure. If you wish to simply make weight loss progress, you will need to adhere to the diet. Your performance will begin to decline if you deviate too far from the diet. If this occurs, simply return to the

2-week protocol and review the basic principles of the diet.

Here are a few quick tips to help you maintain your Bulletproof status while travelling or dining out.

Select a protein. Either wild-caught or raised on grass. If neither of these options is available, opt for chicken or turkey instead. These two foods are low in fat. They contain fewer harmful fats that will be absorbed by the body. Fish caught in the wild and grass-fed cattle are the best sources of fat.

As a side dish, choose a vegetable. Preferably steamed to eliminate any unknown oils that may have been applied.

Pick a lipid. This is the most crucial detail to remember. 70% of your caloric intake should consist of healthy fats. The majority of dining establishments will not carry brain octane oil, XCT oil, or grass-fed butter. But most do have avocados. Request as much avocado as they will permit you to eat. You could add some of your own fat to the meal.

Certain Foods Containing Synthetic Ingredients That Are Killing Us Internally

Over the past couple hundred years, we have stuffed our food with numerous poisonous additives. Now, food additives are substances that are added to food in order to improve its appearance, flavour, or flavour retention. There are natural food additives like salt and vinegar, but these are not the ones that the bulletproof diet opposes. Instead, the bulletproof diet opposes synthetic food additives, some of which are derivatives of natural products and others wholly synthetic. These new food additives contain numerous substances, including artificial sweeteners and food colorings. To prevent food from drying out, humidifiers are added to them. Foods are given a glossy appearance by glazing agents. Emulsifiers prevent the separation of oil and water in homogenised milk, ice creams, mayonnaise, etc., whereas colour retention agents aid in the preservation of food colour. Now, if we consumed these additives in small amounts, they would not be as dangerous; however, our diets are loaded with processed foods, frozen foods, and fast foods that are loaded with these dangerous substances.

Saccharin is used in Sweet n' Low as an artificial sweetener. Numerous studies have demonstrated a link between saccharin and cancer, which calls its safety record into question. Despite FDA approval, you must be cautious about the foods you consume. It is preferable to err on the side of caution and avoid or limit your consumption of these substances than to act irresponsibly and suffer the consequences later on.

Because it has been shown to cause cancer in animals, potassium bromate is another nefarious additive that has been banned everywhere except Japan and the United States. Typically, it is used to increase the volume of bread and rolls.

When monosodium glutamate-sensitive individuals consume products containing this ingredient, they typically experience nausea, vomiting, and severe headaches. Some studies suggest that Monosodium Glutamate and similar additives may also be responsible for rare instances of cardiac arrest. This product is frequently difficult to identify due to the fact that it is frequently disguised as sodium caseinate, textured protein, glutamic acid, glutamate, monopotassium glutamate, autolyzed yeast and other yeast products, gelatin, or calcium caseinate, all of which contain MSG.

High Fructose Corn Syrup and Obesity have an undeniable connection. Researchers from Princeton University demonstrated that rats fed high fructose corn syrup gained significantly more weight than rats that did not consume HFCS, despite the fact that their caloric intake was identical. What does this indicate? High fructose corn syrup should be avoided.

Coca-Cola has decided to eliminate sodium benzoate from its products gradually. Why? Because sodium benzoate, when combined with ascorbic acid or vitamin C, generates benzene, an extremely hazardous carcinogenic compound Sodium Benzoate is used to prevent the growth of fungi and bacteria, but what good is it if it protects you from pathogens but causes cancer? Follow the bulletproof rule and steer clear of sodium benzoate-containing products.

Additionally, sodium nitrite and nitrate are known to increase the risk of cancer. It is used to preserve meats and should also be avoided as much as possible.

Olestra, also known as Olean, is known to cause gastrointestinal issues, abdominal cramps, and to slow or even prevent the absorption of essential vitamins. It is used in fat-free potato chips by the snack food giant Frito Lay.

Some producers add sulphites to their fruits and wines to prevent bacterial growth and fermentation. Some people are allergic to sulphites, and in extremely rare cases, the allergic reaction can be fatal. Although it is not as popular as it once was, it is still present in some products, so you must be cautious about what you consume. The bulletproof diet will increase your awareness and enhance your health.

Banana Pancake

Ingredients:

6 ripe bananas

6 tablespoons almond butter

4 eggs, beaten

6 tablespoons unsalted butter

Direction:

1. Bananas are peeled and mashed with a fork.

2. Add the beaten fresh eggs to the banana purée and thoroughly combine.

3. Add almond butter to the mixture and thoroughly combine.

4. Melt some butter in a pan and add a quarter cup of batter.

5. Easy cook pancakes on each side for about 1-5 minutes.

Serve without delay.fresh eggs Easy cook

Cheesecake Pancakes

Ingredients

1 teaspoon cinnamon

4 fresh eggs

2 teaspoon granulated sugar substitute

4 oz cream cheese

Directions

1. Add all of the ingredients to the blender and blend until the desired consistency is reached.

2. Two minutes are such required for the bubbles to settle.

3. Pour a quarter of the batter into a pan that is hot and well-greased with butter or Pam spray.

4. Just Take approximately two minutes to easy cook until golden brown. Flip and easy cook the opposite side for

an additional minute, then repeat with the remaining batter.

Serve the pancakes with berries and any sugar-free syrup of your choosing.easy cook easy cook simply make Avocado and Mushroom Morning Meal

Ingredients:

- 4 tablespoons grass fed butter or ghee

- Salt to taste

- Pepper powder to taste

- Fresh herbs of your choice to garnish

- 2 medium avocado, peeled, pitted, sliced

- 4 large pastured fresh eggs

- 8 large Portobello mushrooms

- 12 high quality pastured bacon slices

Direction:

1. Easily put a nonstick pan over medium-low heat.

2. Add fifty percent of the butter.

3. Place the mushrooms with their cap facing downward.

4. Sauté until mushrooms are tender. Sprinkle salt and pepper over it.

5. Easily remove from heat and transfer to a platter for serving.

6. Return the pan to the stovetop and add the remaining butter.

7. Add bacon.

8. Crack fresh eggs into the pan and easy cook until done.

9. Transfer to a serving platter.

Serve with slices of avocado.Easily remove easy cook Easily remove

The Breakfast Of Your Dreams On A Budget

Ingredients

500 Grams of brie

20 Eggs

60 Grams of butter

500 Grams of hash browns

400 Grams of bacon

1. Cooking the bacon is the first order of business.

2. While your bacon is cooking, you can easy cook your eggs in a muffin tin.

3. In the muffin hole, you must beat fresh eggs. When the bacon is

finished cooking, set it aside and allow it to cool.

4. I would recommend frying your eggs in bacon fat because they will be crispier and taste better.

5. Simply make sure to cut the bacon into extremely small pieces.

6. Now is the time to sprinkle a bit of bacon over the fresh eggs that have been placed in the muffin cups.

7. Brie will be added as the final ingredient. Be sure to shred your brie cheese before incorporating it into the mixture.

8. You will need to thoroughly combine all of the ingredients, as failure to do so will result in a dish that does not taste as good.

9. The muffin tins must then be placed in the oven and baked at 450 degrees

for approximately 10-20 minutes and six seconds.

When you easily remove the muffin tins from the oven, you are finished. You may wish to use a sandwich bag to keep this food fresh. This meal will last at least three days, and you will no longer need to prepare breakfast every morning. It is reasonable to assume that you can serve this dish with vegetables, and this is a significant consideration. I enjoy serving this dish with chilli and tomato.easy cook simply make simply make

Honey-Café Smoothie

Ingredients

- 3 teaspoon of raw honey

- 5-10 ice cubes

- ¼ cup of brewed Bulletproof Coffee

- 3 cup of raw organic milk of choice

- 2   tablespoon of cocoa powder, unsweetened

Directions

1. Add all of the ingredients together in a small sauce pan.

2. Mix them together until they are warm then add them into a blender with 2 cup of ice.

3. Blend the mixture until it is even and smooth.

Spicy Bacon Wraps

Ingredient List:

• ½ teaspoons of Black Pepper, For Taste

• ½ teaspoons of Garlic, Powdered Variety

• 4 teaspoons of Hot Sauce, Your Favorite Kind

• 1-5 Slices of Bacon, Thick Cut

• 4 Avocados, Fresh, Peeled, Pitted and Cut into Slivers

• ½ teaspoons of Chili, Powdered Variety

Instructions:

1. Wrap each of your avocado slivers with your bacon and place onto a lightly oiled baking sheet.

60

Strawberry-Pineapple Shake

Ingredients:

2 cup coconut milk

1 cup crushed ice

1 cups fresh strawberries

8 slices fresh pineapple

2 cup coconut water

Directions:

1. In a powerful blender or food processor, combine all the ingredients and pulse until smooth and creamy.

2. As it tends to lose nutrients over time, pour the smoothie into glasses and serve as soon as possible.

64

Green Lime

Ingredients:

- ½ cup almonds
- 4 cups Baby spinach
- 12 Juice of limes
- 4 teaspoons grated lime zest
- ˙ 2 cup fresh almond milk

Direction:

1. Lightly steam spinach.
2. Easily put all the ingredients into a blender.
3. Start on a low speed and increase to a high speed.
4. Stop blending when all ingredients are fully blended.

Haddock Fillet With Fennel, Lemon, And Parsley

fresh lemon

Ingredients

Juice of 4 fresh lemons

6 tablespoon coconut oil

Salt and pepper to taste

4 fillets of haddock

4 cups fennel, finely sliced

½ cup flat leaf parsley, chopped

Direction:

1. Place fillets of haddock in bamboo steamer and easy cook for around 8-20 minutes.

2. Add the fennel, fresh lemon juice, parsley and salt and pepper to a bowl with the coconut oil. Mix well.

3. Serve the salad on a plate on top of the haddock fillets.

Spicy Bacon Wraps

Ingredients:

1/2 teaspoon ground black pepper

½ teaspoon garlic powder Hot sauce

20 slices bacon

4 avocados, peeled and pitted.

½ teaspoon chili powder

Method:

1. Wrap each avocado slivers with bacon and place them in a lightly oiled baking sheet.

2. Season the wraps with garlic powder and black pepper.

3. Bake the baking sheet at 350°F for 35 to 40 minutes.

4. Transfer the wraps on a platter and then sprinkle with hot sauce and chili powder before serving.

Baked Burgers

Ingredients:

4 T dried oregano

Sea salt (to taste)

8 slices bacon

4 lbs. ground beef 4 tsp. ground turmeric

2 T dried rosemary

Directions:

1. Preheat oven to 350 degrees F. Make about 8-8 ½ burgers.

2. Combine the spices and rub them directly onto the burgers.

3. Salt to taste.

71

4. Easily put a half-slice of bacon on top of each burger and easily put them on a flat baking pan with sides.

5. Bake for 35 to 40 minutes to desired doneness.

. Sardine Salad

Ingredients:

500g sardines in tomato-based sauce

4 teaspoons Capers, rinsed
1 Cup Black Olives, 2 tablespoons apple cider vinegar
4 tablespoons olive oil
8 cups mixed salad greens

1. In a bowl, whisk olive oil, tomato sauce and apple cider vinegar and then set aside.

2. Easily put the salad greens, black olives and capers in a large bowl.

3. Mix the dressing and the sardines in a bowl.

4. Then, gently mix to combine. Serve immediately.

2 2. Bacon Maple Bulletproof Espresso

Ingredients:

- 2 tsp vanilla extract
- 4 tbsp sugar-free maple syrup
- Whipped cream for topping
- 2 bacon slice, cooked and crumbled

- 2 cup freshly brewed coffee
- 2 tbsp MCT oil
- 2 tbsp butter
- 2 tsp maple extract

1. Add all the ingredients except the whipped cream and bacon to a blender, and process until smooth. Pour the drink into a large glass, swirl some whipped cream on top and garnish with the bacon.

2. Enjoy!

Salmon And Spinach Fresh Eggs

2 teaspoon of herbs of your choice

1 red pepper

900 g frozen spinach with cream

800 g pink salmon

8 fresh eggs

Preparation of Salmon and spinach eggs:

1. Preheat the oven to 250 Degrees.

2. Mix all the ingredients.

3.   Pour into muffin tins, almost to the edge.

4. Bake for about 30 minutes.

Cauliflower Curry

Ingredients:

½ cup water
 2 teaspoon curry powder

 2 head cauliflower
 2 cup coconut milk

1. Rinse cauliflower and pat dry.

2. Trim the cauliflower and separate the   florets.

3. Easily put the florets, cashews, coconut milk and water in a pan and

easy cook over medium heat for about 20 minutes.

4. Easily remove the pan from heat and use a fork to mash the cauliflower.

5. Some   Season it with curry and a pinch of salt before serving.

Smoothie Made With Coconut

Serves: 2

Time: 6 minutes

Ingredients:

- 1 vanilla bean, seeds scraped out

- 1 lemon, zested

- 1 cup coconut full cream milk

- ½ cup filtered water

- 2 tablespoon MCT oil

- 4 tablespoons bulletproof whey protein

Directions:

1. Place all ingredients in a food processor.

2. Pulse until smooth.

3. Serve immediately in a tall glass.

Sweet Bulletproof Egg Salad

Ingredients:

- 3 tablespoon xylitol, stevia, or other bulletproof-approved sweetener

- 15-20 drops vanilla

- 12 fresh egg whites, raw pastured

- 2 scoop bulletproof-approved protein powder

- 2 ounce all-natural chocolate chips

Preparation:

1. Hard boil fresh eggs and chop.

2. Once cooled, combine with remaining ingredients and enjoy!

Fresh Lemon Garlic Creme De Poulet

Fresh lemon 2 cup of milk

1 of a cup of provolone cheese

6 tablesp of olive oil

2 pound of breast of chicken

The juice from one fresh lemon

2 tablesp of mined garlic

1. Heat the oil up in a pan on the stove. Add the garlic and the fresh lemon juice to the oil.

2. Place the chicken in and easy cook on medium high for about 25 to 30 minutes.

3. Once it has finished cooking, add the milk and the provolone cheese.

84

4. Easily Reduce it to a simmer until the mixture begins to get creamy.

5. Stir the chicken up so that it is coated with the creamy mixture.